Exposure Therapy

Orion DiLorenzo

Booky-Books No. 3
RIT Press
Rochester, New York

Published and distributed by:
RIT Press
90 Lomb Memorial Drive
Rochester, New York 14623
https://press.rit.edu

Printed in the United States of America

ISBN 978-1-956313-31-4 (print)

We gather on the traditional territory of the Onöndowa'ga:' or "the people of the Great Hill."
In English, they are known as Seneca people, "the keeper of the western door." They are one of the six nations that make up the sovereign Haudenosaunee Confederacy.
We honor the land on which RIT was built and recognize the unique relationship that the Indigenous stewards have with this land. That relationship is the core of their traditions, cultures, and histories. We recognize the history of genocide, colonization, and assimilation of Indigenous people that took place on this land. Mindful of these histories, we work towards understanding, acknowledging, and ultimately reconciliation.

Designed by Orion DiLorenzo | Cover designed by Marnie Soom

Have you ever gotten a
song stuck in your head?

Maybe a catchy
jingle or tune?

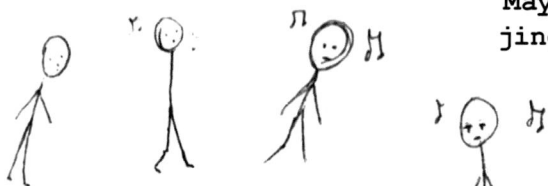

I find myself
listening to
the song in an
attempt to quiet
it down,

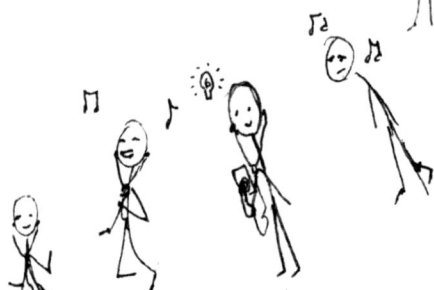

but instead it just feels so
much louder than before.

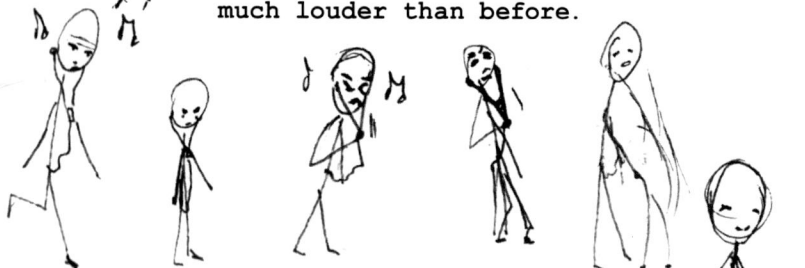

I find myself getting annoyed and
frustrated; it's as if the song will
never get out of my head.

But in the end, the song
leaves my brain and I can
feel at ease.

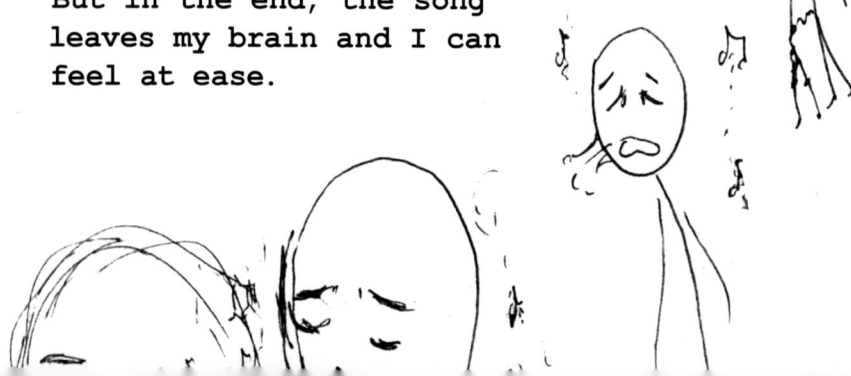

Unlike these songs, which oftentimes are just
annoying, some individuals may experience absurd
and/or terrifying
thoughts that
may leave them
feeling anxious
or afraid.

They're called
"intrusive
thoughts."

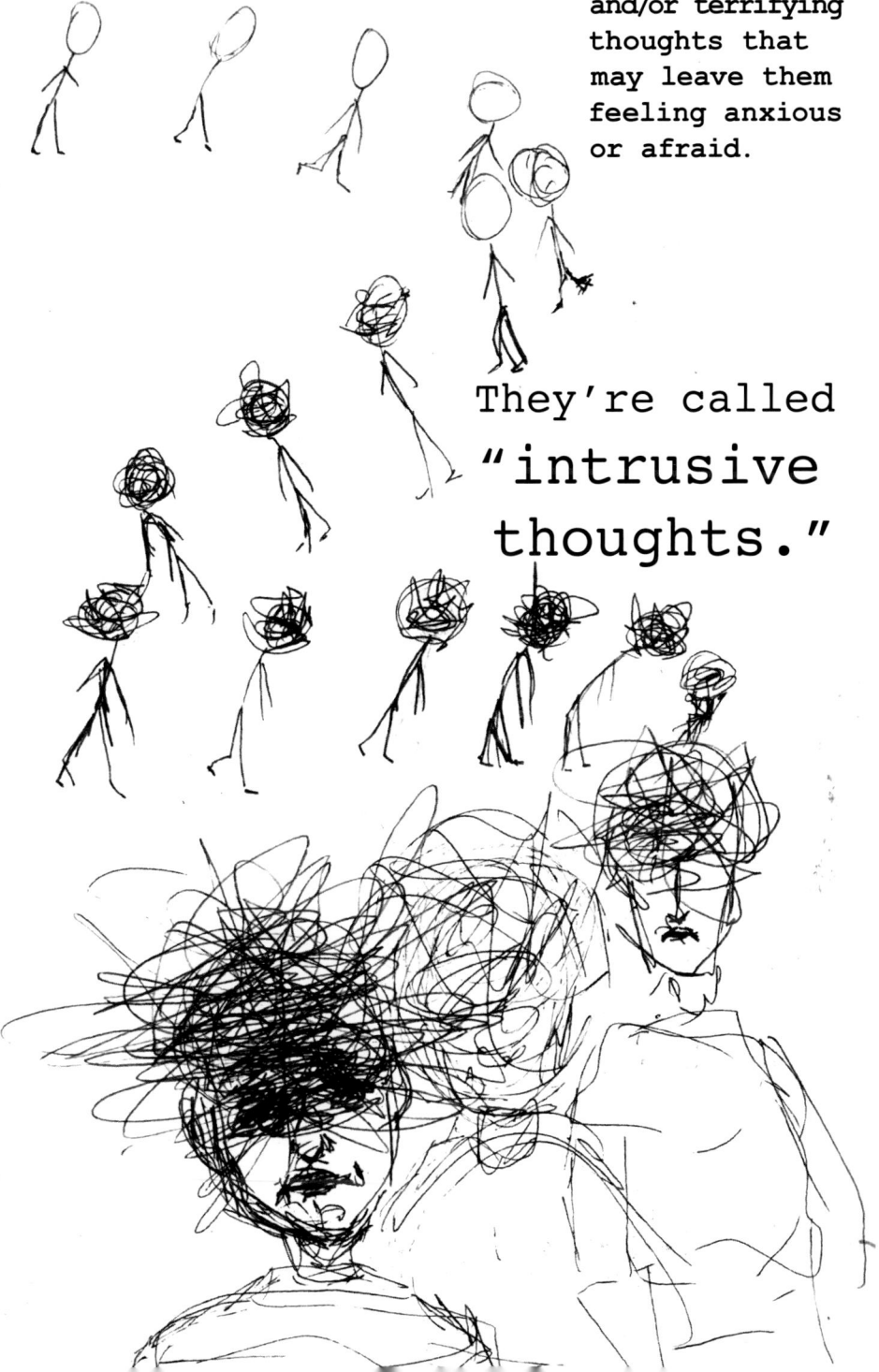

Some examples include:

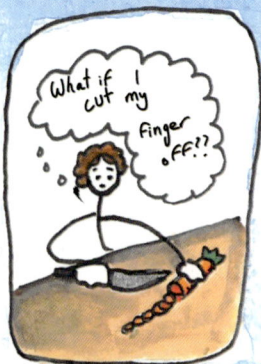

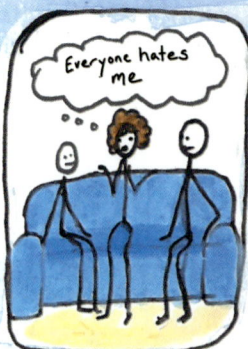

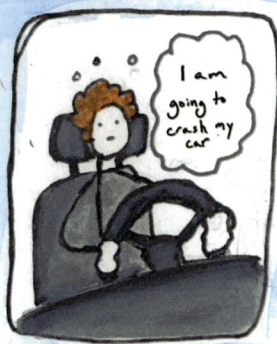

While unpleasant, they are only thoughts and only you can decide what to act on. However, individuals with OCD may experience these thoughts at a higher frequency.

My therapist referenced an OCD workbook multiple times prior to my diagnosis.

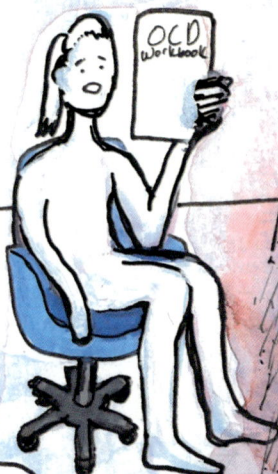

I didn't accept it at first; I had a deep misunderstanding of obsessions and compulsions.

I only sought help when I saw that my fears could potentially harm my relationship with my friend.

In the spring of 2024, I made a new friend, Kovu. He was great to game with and really funny.

He was also the first Black friend of mine to frequently use the n-word.

Like an earworm, the word dug its way into my brain and played on repeat. I hated it. I felt as if the word was on the tip of my tongue like a ticking time bomb.

I did not tell Kovu my fears. I was afraid of him thinking poorly of me for even thinking the word.

If I said anything vaguely resembling the n-word (such as vinegar), I'd end up repeating the word over and over again.

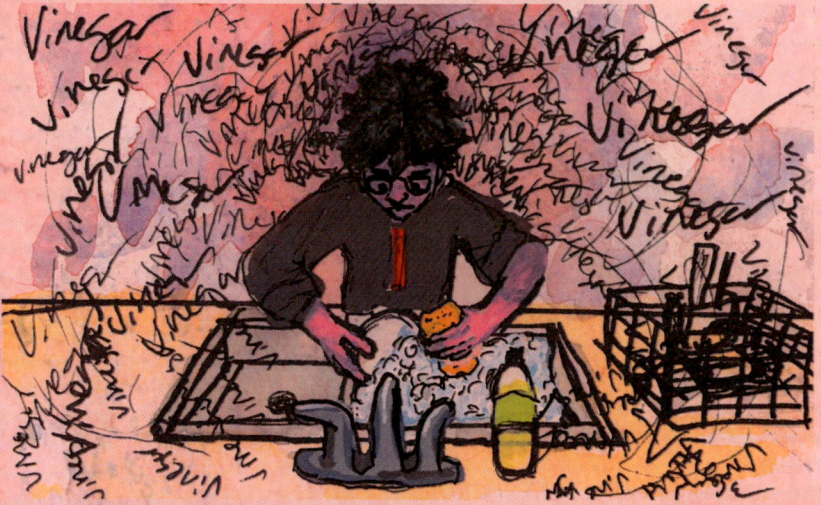

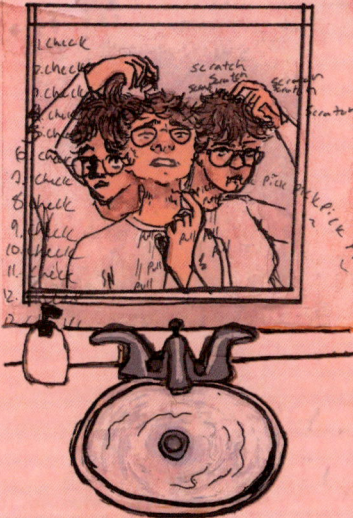

When the thoughts got really loud, I'd find myself standing in front of the mirror, scratching, checking, and picking my scalp or the bumps on my skin.

These compulsions provided me temporary relief.

However, the relief was always short-lived. The thoughts would come back and so would the compulsions. I couldn't focus in class, I struggled to talk to my loved ones, and I was always resisting the urge to pull my hair out.

I don't remember exactly what happened.

One night when I was really tired, I searched online,

"fear of blurting out obscenities." All the results were OCD related.

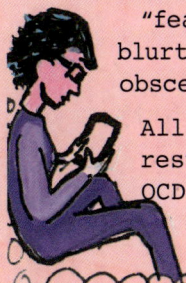

Oh shit frfr??

When I mentioned this to my therapist, she pulled out the OCD booklet again

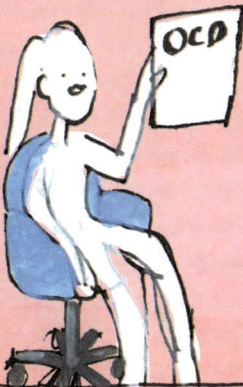

OCD

This time, I accepted it.

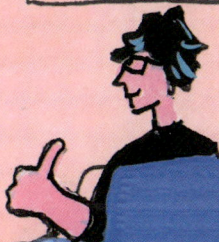

I've printed out some resources for you.

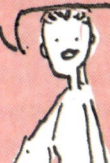

You can also email me with any questions.

What is OCD?

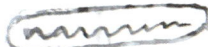

We'll prep for exposure therapy next week.

Exposure therapy??

Huh?

Expose me to what???

Will I have to say the n-word???

No... That can't be right.... Right?

I had no idea what to expect.

Something no one tells you about getting an OCD diagnosis is the amount of paperwork you have to do.

First up: The Yale—Brown Obsessive—Compulsive Scale

It's a long and confusing process.

I think I redid this 3 times?

I kept misinterpreting the examples.

AGGRESSIVE OBSESSIONS

Past	Current		Example
	X	I fear I might harm myself	Fear of handling sharp objects, [...]
	X	I fear I might harm others	Fear of pushing someone in front of a train, fear of hurting someone's feelings [...]
	X	I fear I will blurt out obscenities	Fear of shouting obscenities in public situations [...]
	X	I fear doing something embarrassing	Fear of appearing foolish in social situations
		I have horrific ... in my	Images of murder. dis...

CHECKING COMPULSIONS

Past	Current		Example
	X	I check that I did not harm myself	Checking that you haven't hurt someone without knowing it. You may ask others for reassurance [...]
	X	I check that I did not harm others	Checking that you have 't hurt someone without knowing it [...]
		I check that I did not make a mistake	Repeated checking of door locks, stoves, electrical outlets, before leaving [...]
		I check tha* ...	...e for news about ... he that you

TIME OCCUPIED BY OBSESSIVE THOUGHTS

	0 =	None
	1 =	Less than 1 hour per day, or occasional intrusions (occur no more than 8 times a day)
	2 =	1-3 hours per day, or frequent intrusions (most of the day are free of obsessions
X	3 =	More than 3 hours and up to 8 hours per da , or very frequent intrusions
	4 =	More than 8 hours per day; near-constant intrusions

It helped my therapist and I determine my obsessions and compulsions and their severities.

Based on that list, I ranked situations that made me feel the most anxious. Rather than start with the scariest situations, I'd tackle the bottom of the ranking and move upward.

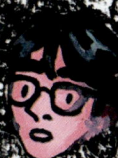

"SUDS" rating
Subjective Units of Distress Scale

Anxiety Provoking Situation	SUDS (0-100)
Eating steak	100
Accidentally saying the n-word	90
Saying something mean to others	80
Cutting Veggies w/ Joan in the kitchen	60
Eating gummy worms	50
Saying "I'm uncomfortable"	40

For each exposure exercise, I had to avoid compulsions and note my distress. When the SUDS rating halved, I'd move on to a new exercise.

Exposure exercise: Eating a gummy worm

Compulsions or responses to avoid: pocketing food in mouth, no cutting food in half, no checking to see if I'm choking, no spitting

Date	Exposure Length	SUDS rating Start of exercise	SUDS rating End of exercise	Notes
4/21 10:32 am	1 minute	20	0	3 gummy bears
12:18 4/24	3 minutes	30	0	1 gummy worm was hard to not do a compulsion
12:25 4/26	3 minutes	40	0	I did not do any compulsions. I am ok!
12:38 4/30	2 minutes	10	0	

These tasks may seem mundane... and they are!

Eat 3 gummy worms

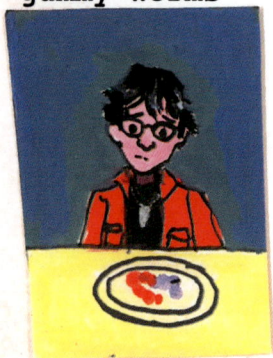

Hold a knife for 10 minutes

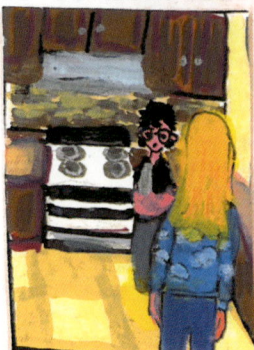

Practice saying, "I'm uncomfortable"

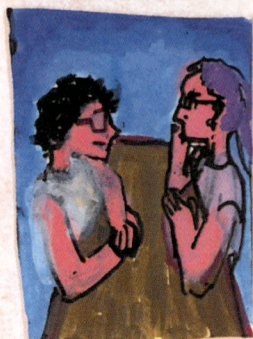

OCD is debilitating in that way; it makes everyday tasks feel impossible. These tasks helped me gain the courage to take my life back.

Fears that could potentially harm others, such as saying a racial slur, are tackled through "imaginative exercises" where you walk through a potential scenario. I learned that I will not blurt out anything I don't want to say, and if I somehow do, I can apologize and talk to others about what's going on in my brain.

I am not a horrible person for having these thoughts —

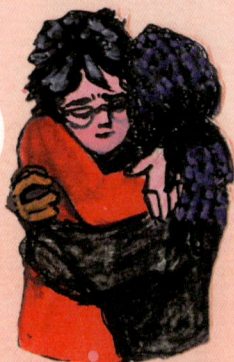

just a person struggling with OCD.

I never ended up performing any imaginary exercises, though.

The night I got diagnosed, I called Kovu to tell him my fear of blurting out the n-word.

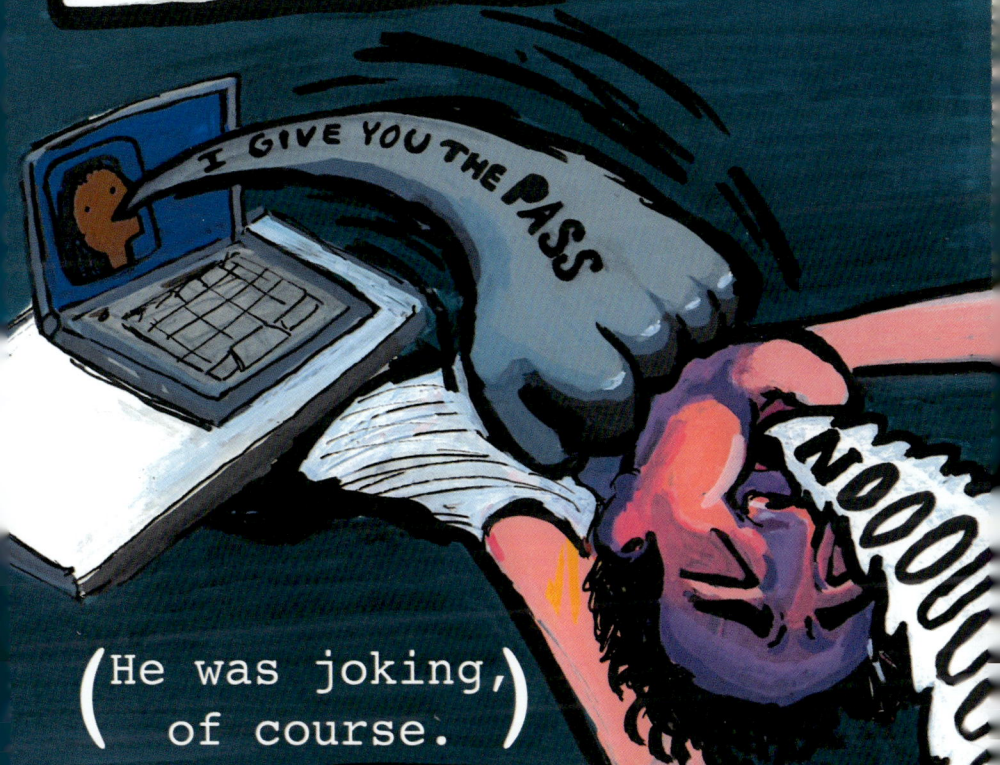

I GIVE YOU THE PASS

NOOOOOOOO

(He was joking,) of course.

I don't know what I was expecting... Disgust? Anger? Confusion? I never considered that Kovu wouldn't be hate me for my thoughts — let alone immediately make a joke about it. Further discussion showed me how kind and understanding he was. By talking about my fear, I finally understood how absurd it was. This newfound relief led me to begin opening up to my loved ones again and talking freely.

Kovu, our friends, and I went on a road trip to Canada.

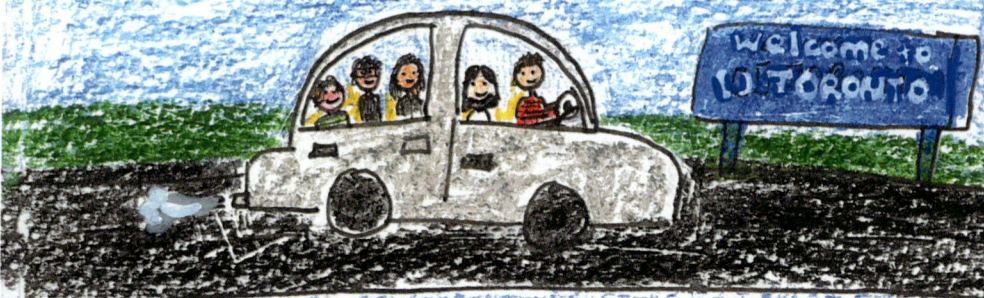

Welcome to TORONTO

It was a long, chatty car ride, so deep conversations and stories from our past kept popping up.

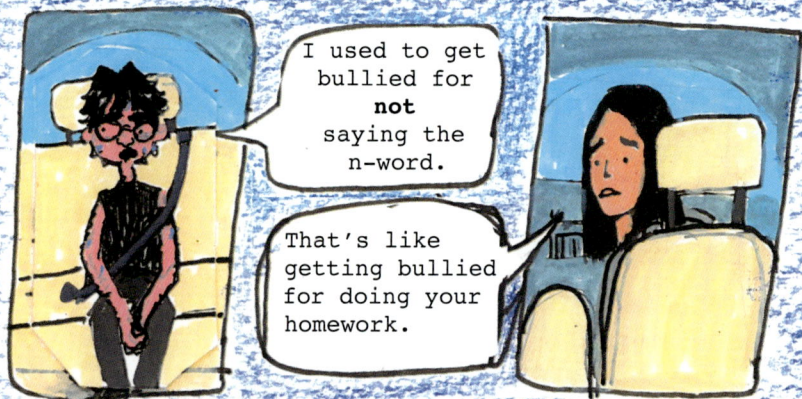

I used to get bullied for **not** saying the n-word.

That's like getting bullied for doing your homework.

Around 2013, many of my peers would try to emulate their favorite rappers at the time by using African American Vernacular English and slurs. When I voiced discomfort, they would say that I was a buzzkill and annoying. One person in particular took joy in antagonizing me by repeatedly saying it in my ear.

I never shared my experiences before that car ride with my friends. I was afraid that being in proximity to those people meant I was tainted as well.

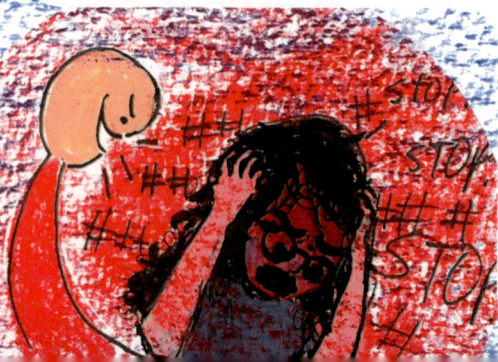

The ugly part of OCD is that some part of me felt that my obsession was "right"; it prevented me from getting help. I climbed up high onto a moral pedestal in an attempt to separate myself from my peers. High up on my pedestal, I felt constant distress over the fear of falling off. I avoided making any mistakes, but how can I learn without failure?

Stepping down from this pedestal meant accepting that I am no better than my peers. We deal with the cards dealt to us to us, and while some of my bullies may still hold their racist beliefs, I know others may regret their past behaviors.

Rather than agonizing over avoiding harm, I can instead take the time to learn how to heal any wounds I cause.

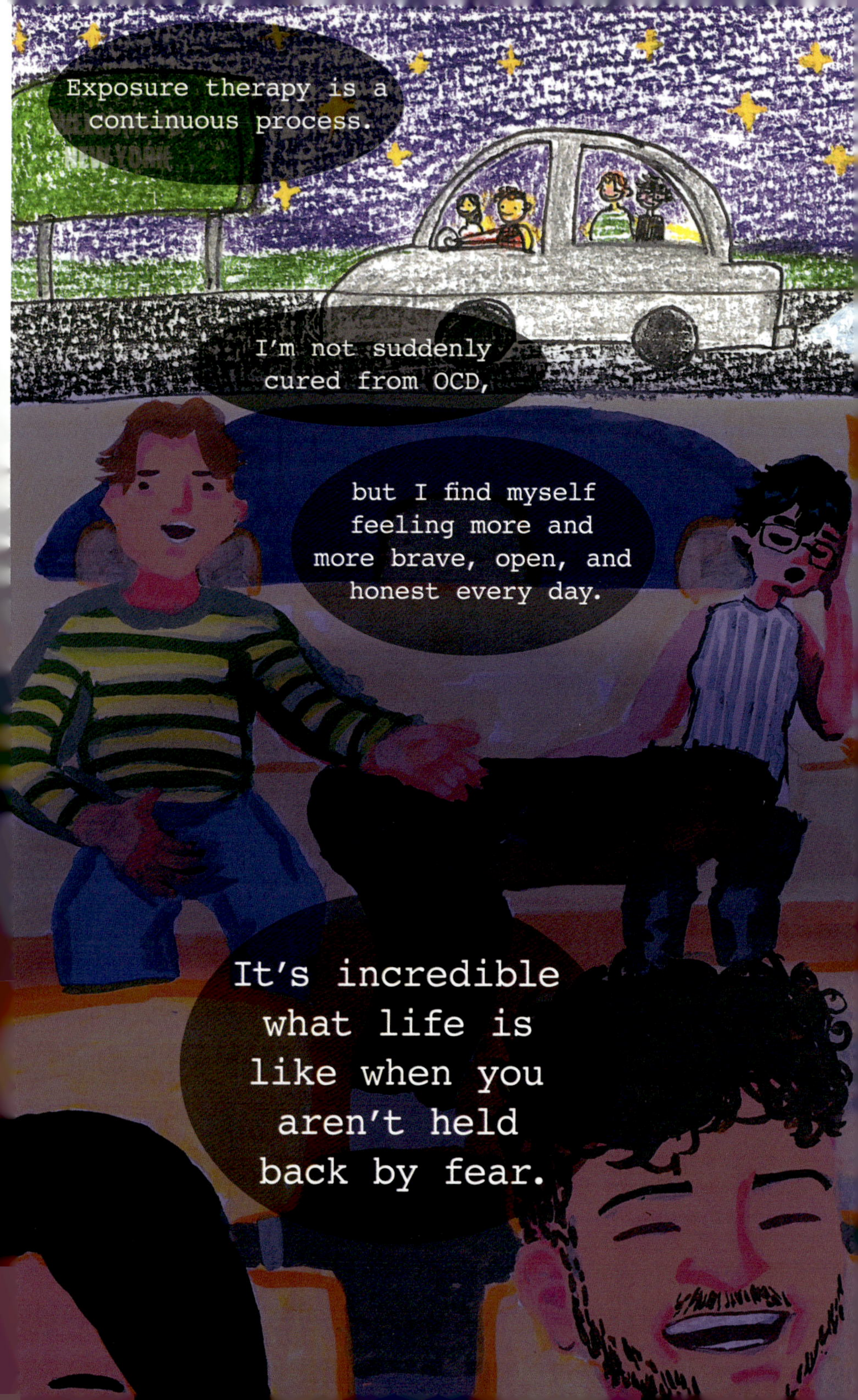
Exposure therapy is a continuous process.
I'm not suddenly cured from OCD,
but I find myself feeling more and more brave, open, and honest every day.
It's incredible what life is like when you aren't held back by fear.

Exposure therapy is a treatment
used for OCD, anxiety, phobias,
and more.

If you are struggling with mental
health, please reach out to a
licensed mental health professional.

Mental Health Resources:
CDC Resources:
www.cdc.gov/mental-health/caring

International OCD foundation:
www.iocdf.org

Works Cited:

Goodman, W. K., Price, L. H., Rasmussen, S.
A., Mazure, C., Fleischmann, R. L., Hill, C.
L., Heninger, G. R., & Charney, D. S. (1989).
Yale-Brown Obsessive Compulsive Scale (YBOCS)
[Database record]. APA PsycTests.
https://doi.org/10.1037/t57982-000

Orion Dilorenzo is a computer
science major at RIT. Inspired by
their hometown of Monmouth Beach,
New Jersey, they can be found
presenting "Funny Fish Friday"
every Friday at the Society of
Software Engineers. On Wednesdays,
they can be found giving technical
art talks as RITGraph's vice
president. Every day, they can be
found doodling something new.

At home, they're a proud parent to
Shallot the Crested Gecko, October
the Fire Skink, and a little rat
dog named Mila.

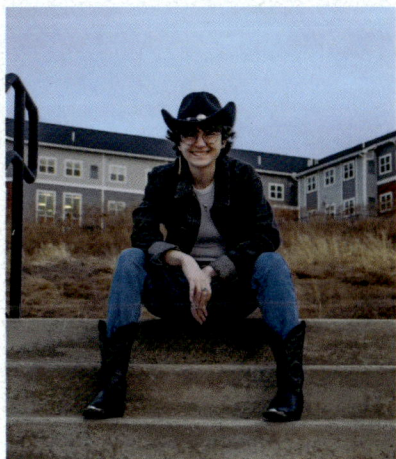

Instagram: @mikufan79

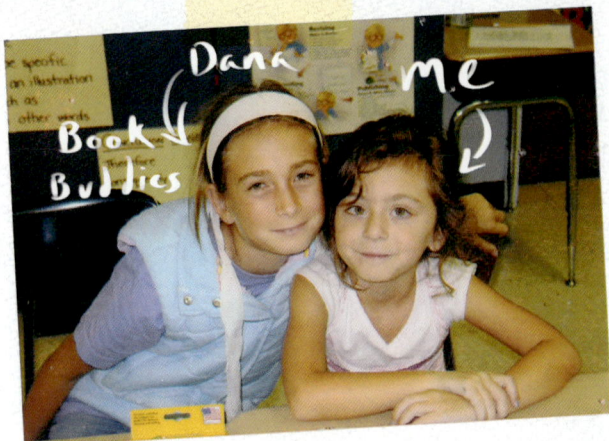
Dana
me
Book
Buddies

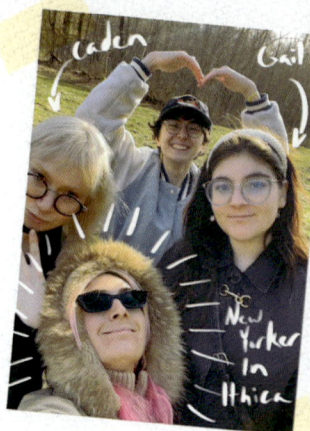
caden
Gail
New Yorker In Ithica

In Loving Memory of:
Dana "Lioness" Wiener

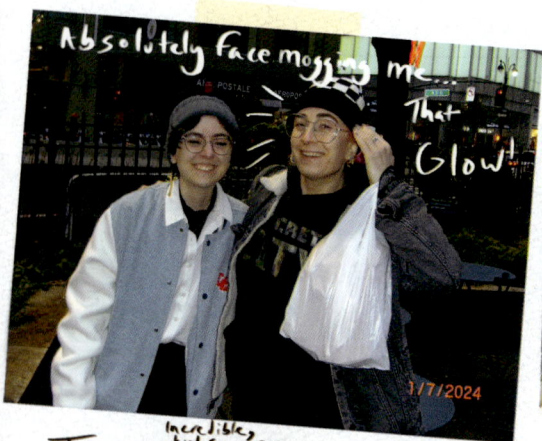
Absolutely face mogging me...
That Glow!
1/7/2024

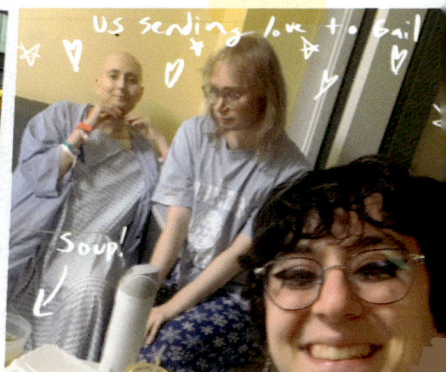
Us sending love to Gail
Soup!

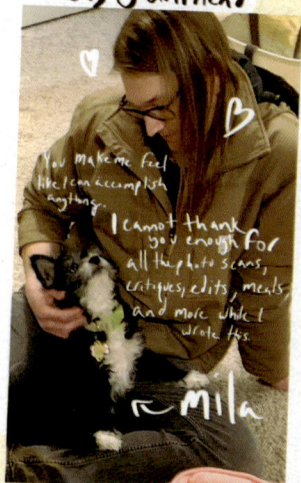
Joan, my Girlfriend
Incredibly kind, smart, funny,
♡
You make me feel like I can accomplish anything.
I cannot thank you enough for all the photo scans, critiques, edits, meals, and more while I write this.
~mila

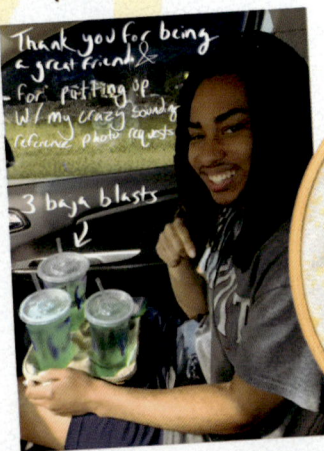
Kovu
Thank you for being a great friend & for putting up w/ my crazy sounding reference photo requests.
3 baja blasts

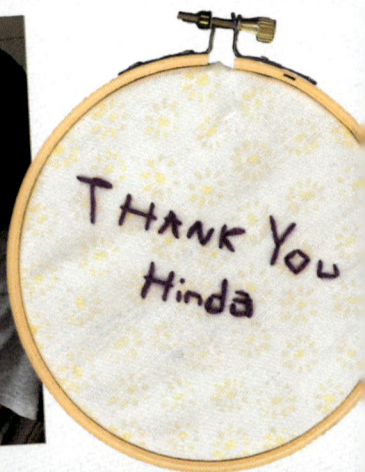
THANK YOU
Hinda